What sh...

A Handy Gu...
Irritable Bo...

Text:

... *..y of Manchester*

Dr Andrew Robinson,
*Clinical Lecturer in Gastroenterology –
University of Manchester*

Paul Buckley, *Writer*

Illustrations:	John Whatmore
Design:	Sid Carter
First edition:	May 2000 2,000 copies
UK publishers:	RTFB Publishing Limited, Building 2, Shamrock Quay, Southampton SO14 5QL
For more information:	Phone (023) 8022 9041 Fax (023) 8022 7274

Acknowledgements
Patients with IBS who gave time to share their experiences of the condition. Thank you for your enthusiasm and support.

Consultants and staff at Hope Hospital, Salford.

© The University of Manchester 2000

'What should I do?' is the copyright of Ketting Partners BV and its logo is used with the permission of the copyright holder and its UK licensee - RTFB Publishing Limited.

ISBN 1 902983 11 4

NATIONAL PRIMARY CARE RESEARCH AND DEVELOPMENT CENTRE

THE UNIVERSITY *of* MANCHESTER

An Mpower publication

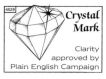

Crystal Mark

Clarity approved by Plain English Campaign

This guidebook has gained Plain English Campaign's Crystal Mark

Contents

Introduction: What this book is for

Introduction

Irritable bowel syndrome

What do the words mean?

Irritable: the bowel is very sensitive to normal digestive events and overreacts to them.

Bowel: the colon or large intestine.

Syndrome: a group of symptoms which describes a condition.

Clear and thorough information about an illness such as irritable bowel syndrome (IBS) is important. It can help people to understand what is happening to them so that they can cope with the symptoms and the effect IBS has on their everyday lives. Good information lets people know the different treatments that are available and will help them to make the most of the limited time they have with their GP and other NHS health professionals.

There are a number of sources of information which you may find helpful. Information about the disease based on medical and nursing evidence is very important in understanding the medical problem and finding out about the best types of treatment that are available from the health services. However, ordinary people who have experience of living with IBS every day have other forms of knowledge which may be just as important in helping you to learn to live with and manage your illness.

Knowledge based on people's experience is not often acknowledged. Research into the way people experience illness suggests that people who have gone through the various phases of an illness know what the personal and social results of the illness are, and, over time, they become experts in understanding and responding to a particular illness. IBS is likely to affect people's lives, their relationships with others, their work and leisure activities. Because of their experience and knowledge, people with IBS are in a very good position to help others who are in a similar position. They know what it is like trying to discuss things with health professionals and what help to expect from these contacts.

People have their own theories about what causes IBS, and these theories deserve to be recognised as valid possibilities because the medical cause is still uncertain. People who have had IBS have usually tried a range of treatments and remedies and have often developed their own ways of coping. Health professionals may not be well informed about how people experience and manage their IBS, so it is important to let others know what you do and do not find useful.

The information in this guide tries to combine evidence from medical professionals and people with IBS to provide people with a resource which we hope will be useful to them.

Anne Rogers
Professor of the Sociology of Health Care
University of Manchester

Chapter 1
Personal experiences of IBS

"A good set of bowels is worth more to a man than any quantity of brains." **Josh Billings**

This guide was written with the help of people who have irritable bowel syndrome (IBS). Several groups of people with IBS met to talk about their problems and decide what sort of information they would find most helpful. The quotes in this guide are from people with IBS who came to those meetings. Everyone who came to the meetings agreed that talking about their IBS helped them a great deal. What they really wanted to know was how other people managed their lives. This first chapter will introduce you to other people who live with IBS. You will probably find you have many similar feelings and experiences and hopefully it will show you that you are not alone.

Many people have IBS. It is difficult to give exact numbers because a lot of people do not consult their doctor, but it is thought that as many as one in two people may have symptoms of IBS at some time in their life. The symptoms come and go, and most people struggle to cope with them.

People with IBS have a gut that does not work properly. We do not know what causes IBS, but we do know some things make it worse. It is a condition that affects people in many ways. This guide aims to give advice which, hopefully, will help you control your IBS symptoms. Some people need help from a GP to find a medicine or diet to control their symptoms. A few people will need help from a specialist gastroenterologist.

All of us find talking about bowel problems embarrassing. IBS can be a lonely and worrying experience.

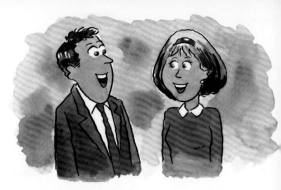

'It is not a serious illness, but it's such a complicated illness. A huge organ that's gone haywire and there doesn't seem to be any cure.'

'The big thing is to find out that it is a proper illness, you know, it's not something I've dreamt up. I think it helps to know there are other people.'

Because there are so many parts to the bowel, people with IBS have many symptoms. They can include constipation, diarrhoea and pain. You may always have the same symptoms, or you may find that your symptoms change. Most of the time, for most people, IBS symptoms will not cause serious problems.

'I can go ... a month, two months and I seem to be ticking over fine and then all of a sudden ... I start with severe constipation then, the griping pains and going to the toilet. The following day I feel as though somebody's jumped all over me.'

'I don't get constipated at all. I go every day but I don't feel like I've been to the toilet when I've been. I still feel my belly's out here.'

'It probably flares up two or three times a year. I tend to have a lot of looseness, bloatedness and nausea.'

'Just like period pains, I roll on the floor and I'm bloated and oh, the wind is appalling.'

'It has side effects, not only your pain - you're bloated, it makes you feel lethargic. I get headaches.'

'You just feel like a piece of lettuce. It just drains you.'

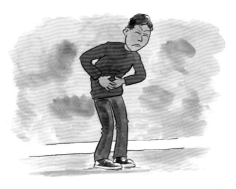

People have quite similar feelings and worries when they have bowel problems.

'I was initially concerned I'd got bowel cancer, the pain was so horrendous, I was convinced there was something seriously wrong, and I had this colonoscopy and they didn't find anything.'

'I find it quite hard to believe, it can just suddenly come like that and you can't get rid of it. There must be something you can do to manage it better, mustn't there?'

One of the problems with IBS is the loss of control people feel.

'It's so unpredictable. One minute you're fine and the next minute it triggers off.'

'I find the toilets before I go anywhere. I've just got to know where the toilets are.'

'I find I can't plan driving any distances if I've got it. I wouldn't attempt to drive more than down to the local supermarket.'

'When I go out, I'm carrying boxes, like pads and wipes because sometimes I just don't have any warning.'

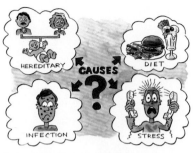

Nobody knows what causes IBS, and not knowing what causes an illness can be frustrating and frightening. For most people, but not everyone, it is very strongly linked to stress. Whether or not stress is the cause, IBS is likely to get worse if you are in a stressful situation.

'I think stress can bring it on with me. I have problems at work, I can get really wound up - that can start it with me.'

'I know when my lad has a fit, I panic and I get all het up and I feel sick and then the next day, toilet all day.'

'I used to get more wound up, I think trying to prove myself. I'm more at peace with myself these days - so whether that's helped to pan it out a bit with me...'

For some people, stress does not seem to be the cause of IBS.

'I seem to get it when I relax, so this idea of stress, I don't think it's really right.'

Some people link the start of IBS to other causes.

'There was a pill scare and I changed my pill - it started after that. It could be hormonal, that could have triggered it off.'

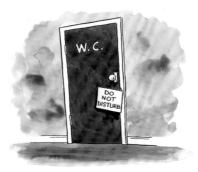

Food and diet are closely linked to IBS. Nearly everyone with IBS knows a food which gives them symptoms. Sometimes, one bad food experience can definitely be linked to the start of IBS.

'As I was eating this turkey I thought "Oh God" it had a very strong taste. The next day I started to be ill, I was ill for a full week. It cleared up, but it's never gone, it's come back and back.'

'I just stop off things like salad and fruit if it's bad. You just learn from experience, you think "Well I'm not having that again" when I'm feeling bloated.'

People find many ways of coping with the problems IBS brings. Some people can cope and manage their IBS on their own.

'I first had the symptoms nearly 25 years ago and I've been through everything the doctor could offer me. I finally worked out a solution myself by changing my diet, that solved the problem for me.'

For most people, IBS will get better over time. This may be because you learn more about how your body reacts to food or to stressful situations. You find ways to cope with these.

'As I've got older, it's more controllable.'

'Slowly, it's not as bad as it was at the beginning.'

'*I think self-help goes a long way. You've got to be realistic and think "Well, what's causing this?" and think of a way round it.*'

Something else that seems to help some people is talking about the problem. IBS is a very common condition. It is very likely that other people you work with or are friends with suffer from IBS too.

'*When I started work there and found all the people who've got it, I was very surprised, but it does help to talk to other people.*'

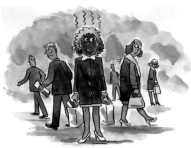

IBS does cause problems and disruptions to your life. Research has found that it is one of the most common reasons people give for taking time off work.

'*I nearly lost this job. Every time I was off and I took a note for IBS, they had me in the office because I was working where there was food. It was very embarrassing, they sat there firing questions at me. I just said I have to keep going to the toilet, I'm not dirty, everybody has to go to the toilet, I just go more often.*'

It often causes problems in your social life too.

'*I remember once I was going to a wedding. I was wearing a very slim fitting skirt with a blouse tucked in. I was in absolute agony. The skirt looked horrendous because my stomach was out here. I was in dreadful pain all night, I couldn't eat any of the buffet.*'

'Last month I went to town. I went to the toilet in a large department store, big queue, I messed myself. I had to go and buy a track suit bottom. I got to my daughter's and I couldn't tell her, I felt that upset. I cleaned myself down and I thought, I wonder if people can smell you. It really gets to you.'

'I haven't had a holiday for three years because of the state of my stomach.'

Other people can seem to be quite unfeeling. This can make you feel terrible.

'One of my neighbours was pregnant early this summer and she said "You're about the same size as me aren't you?" Well, I could've just died of embarrassment 'cos our bumps were very very similar.'

People will have many sorts of experiences with doctors. People who have had IBS for some time generally find they have tried everything their doctors have suggested and try to cope on their own.

'I've not been to my GP for ages. I feel there's nothing they can tell me that I don't know already and that I've not tried already.'

'The doctor said to me "There is not a cure for IBS. You have to learn to manage it." And I do think they are right.'

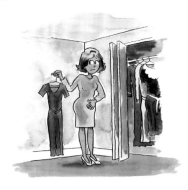

Some people rely on their doctor to give them emotional support. Certain doctors are able to do this, others are not. It can be very upsetting if you do not feel you can talk through your problem with your doctor. You may feel better if you can talk to someone else such as a counsellor or someone who has experienced IBS.

'If you've got somebody who's sympathetic, who knows all about it and who smiles instead of thinking "next", you know, it's really good.'

'Sometimes I talk about it and I burst out crying and the doctor just looks at me, I bet he thinks, "Oh she's here again" and I feel like saying - "please, somebody help me, just give me a bit of a life."'

'It's when they say "It's all in your mind", that's one of the things that really gets me, I think, "Well, it's not, it's in my stomach really."'

'Doctors are not the same as counsellors, you need to sit and talk it through with somebody who listens to what you're thinking about, not just going in and thinking you're gonna get tablets or something.'

'You need a consultant with irritable bowel. That's the answer.'

Things to remember

● A lot of people have IBS.

● You can have many different symptoms.

● IBS is not a serious condition, but it can be hard to cope with.

Chapter 2
Understanding IBS

This chapter will tell you what is known about IBS and about normal digestion. It will explain recent research into IBS.

What is irritable bowel syndrome?

IBS has been known about for a long time. It has been called different things such as: mucus colitis, spastic colitis, spastic colon, irritable colon, nervous diarrhoea, nervous stomach, abdominal migraine and grumbling appendix.

Between 10% and 65% of the population has IBS, the exact number of people is not known because there are many definitions of IBS.

As many as 5% to 10% of the population consult their GP every year for IBS symptoms. IBS is a combination of abdominal pain and a changing bowel habit. It is due to a bowel which does not contract normally and which is very sensitive to any contractions that happen.

Females are three times more likely than males to have IBS. It usually starts in the late teens but it can start at any age.

When people with IBS are examined, their bowels look healthy and blood tests do not show anything unusual. But their bowels still don't work properly.

Some people are pleased to know that tests show nothing is seriously wrong with their body. Other people find the news that 'there is nothing wrong' very frustrating and want a clear physical cause. Research has shown that IBS does **not** lead to cancer.

What do doctors mean by the word 'syndrome'?

A syndrome is a group of symptoms which describe a condition. To diagnose IBS a doctor needs to know if you have two or three of the following symptoms.

- Abdominal pain.

- Diarrhoea.

- Constipation.

- Wind.

- Bloating.

- Feeling you have not completely emptied your bowels.

- Passing mucus.

In many cases, you may have pain after you have eaten, and this is often relieved by opening the bowels.

These are **not** symptoms of IBS:

- passing blood; or

- losing weight.

If you notice either of these symptoms, you must see your doctor as soon as possible because they could be symptoms of bowel disease or bowel cancer. If you are over the age of 40 and have any symptoms of IBS for the first time, you should see your GP who may want to arrange for further tests.

If you are passing blood or have lost more than half a stone without dieting, your doctor may want to send you for tests to rule out a more serious bowel problem.

Medical research

Medical research is done to find out the following things about a condition.

- The number of people who have the condition and whether it is getting more common.

- The type of people who get the condition.

- What symptoms the condition causes.

- What is abnormal in the bodies of people with the condition.

- What makes the symptoms better or worse.

- How safe the treatments are.

We can answer these questions for IBS by talking to patients with the condition, examining the bowel to see if there are any abnormalities and by testing new treatments using clinical trials.

So far, research has shown that there are no clear physical differences between patients with IBS and people who do not have the condition. Many clinical trials have been carried out, looking at different types of treatment.

Clinical trials have been used to test various drugs, psychotherapy, hypnotherapy and complementary therapies. Many studies have unclear results and often involve patients with very specific symptoms for example, they may only include people who have symptoms of constipation. It is difficult to make any general conclusions, but there is no evidence that a single treatment is useful for all people with IBS.

Good research studies are expensive and it is often difficult to get money for research into certain medical conditions. However, medical research has led to a number of theories or ideas about what might be going on. The next sections will show you some of the research that has been done to try and find out more about IBS and its causes.

Theory number 1

Something in what you have eaten may make your gut react badly. Is it an infection? Is it a food intolerance because your body lacks a special chemical? Is it our modern diet? Is it an allergic reaction?

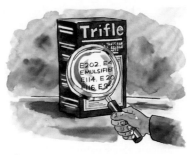

The research

Some research has shown there is a link between people who use a lot of antibiotics throughout their life and IBS. Studies have shown that at least a quarter of people who visit their doctor with IBS have had gastroenteritis before the symptoms began. In these cases, symptoms usually go away after a year. There is strong research evidence that some people who are diagnosed with IBS may have lactose intolerance, so they only get IBS symptoms when they eat or drink dairy products. There is little evidence to show that food allergy is a cause of IBS symptoms.

Theory number 2

There is a theory that the recent increases in food intolerance may be related to a decrease in our exposure to bacteria. Modern homes in Western parts of the world, like the UK, are much cleaner than they used to be. We use a lot more antiseptic and disinfecting solutions to clean our homes and this may be linked to the rise in reports of people who are 'allergic' to the modern world. It might be that the human body needs to be exposed to many types of bacteria early in life to stay healthy. There is no good research evidence to support this theory, but there is no research evidence to say that it is not true.

Theory number 3

People with IBS may have a colon where the muscles do not contract properly. People who have constipation may have a colon where there are not enough muscle contractions. People who have diarrhoea may have a colon where the muscles contract too often.

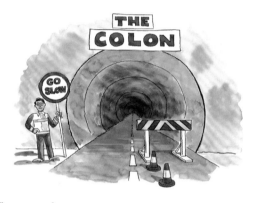

The research

Research on the muscles of the gut involves measuring the changes in pressure inside the gut. This can be done over several hours while people carry on with normal activities wearing the special equipment needed to record the changes in pressure. Some research shows that there are differences between the number and strength of muscle contractions between:

  people who have IBS with constipation;

  people who have IBS with diarrhoea; and

  healthy volunteers.

We still do not know what causes these differences.

Theory number 4

There may be something wrong with the way the gut senses or understands what is happening as food passes through it. This means that the gut does not react normally, leading to the symptoms of IBS. The gut does have its own nervous system which is linked to the brain.

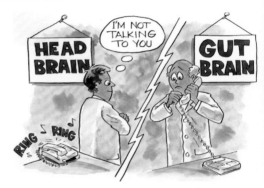

The research

Research has shown that some people with IBS have a hypersensitive gut. Studies where special balloons are put into the gut show that people with IBS feel any changes in pressure much more easily than people who do not have IBS. Recent research has looked at the nerve connections from the gut to the brain and at the way the brain reacts to what is going on in the gut. Results also show that our emotions can affect the sensations we get from the gut.

Theory number 5

Emotional problems may cause gut problems. This happens to everyone. We all get 'butterflies' in our tummy before a stressful event like an exam or an interview and a lot of people get diarrhoea or vomit. Maybe in people with IBS, the emotional link to the gut is stronger.

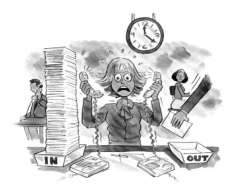

The research

IBS has been shown to be one of the physical ways
the body reacts to stress. Other physical symptoms of
stress include tension headaches, poor resistance to
colds and viral illnesses and high blood pressure.
Researchers have found a clear link between stressful
events and symptoms of IBS.

Theory number 6

IBS might be linked to hormones. It is known that
more women than men are diagnosed with IBS.

The research

There is research which shows that symptoms of
diarrhoea and constipation are linked to the menstrual
cycle. Women with IBS have been found to have more
problems with these symptoms during menstruation
than women who do not have IBS. Hormones which
are at high levels on the first day of a period are
known to make the muscles of the colon contract
more.

It may be that the cause of IBS is due to some, none or
a combination of these six theories.

How does the digestive system work?

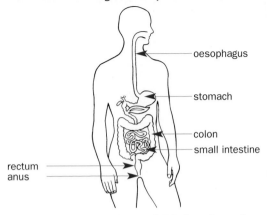

It may help you to understand IBS if you know how the digestive system works.

The gastrointestinal or digestive tract is a hollow tube that goes from the mouth to the anus. It digests food, and nutrients are absorbed through the wall of the gut into the blood stream. Substances such as saliva, mucus and enzymes are passed into the gut to help digest and move food. Digestion is the process that breaks down food and drink into their smallest parts called nutrients. The body uses nutrients to build and nourish cells and to provide energy. Digestion begins in the mouth, when we chew and swallow, and ends in the small intestine. Everything that is not digested ends up in the colon (large intestine).

From the mouth, food passes down the oesophagus into the stomach where it is broken down and digested. Then the food passes into the small intestine. The small intestine is about 6.5 metres (20 feet) long and is called small because the tube is narrower here. Most food is digested and absorbed in the small intestine which has three sections: the duodenum, the jejunum and the ileum.

The ileum joins to the colon. The colon is about

1.5 metres (four feet) long and is called the large intestine because the tube is wide. The colon connects the small intestine with the rectum and anus. In the colon, water is reabsorbed into the blood and the food waste is made into solid stools (faeces). About two litres of liquid goes into the colon from the small intestine each day. This liquid may stay there for hours or days, during which time most of the fluid and salts are absorbed into the body. The stool passes through the colon and into the rectum where it is stored until you go to the toilet.

The hollow organs of the digestive system contain muscles which move the walls of the bowel by contracting and relaxing.

The movement of organ walls pushes food and liquid through the digestive system and can also mix the contents inside each organ. This movement of the oesophagus, stomach, and intestine is called peristalsis. The action of peristalsis is like an ocean wave moving through the muscle. The muscle of the organ narrows and the narrowing is continued slowly down the length of the organ. These waves of narrowing push the food and fluid in front of them through each hollow organ. Muscles of the colon move the contents slowly backwards and forwards, but mainly toward the rectum. A few times each day strong muscle contractions move down the colon pushing faeces ahead of them. Some of these strong contractions make you need to go to the toilet.

The connection between the brain and the gut
The digestive organs receive nerve fibres from the brain and the spinal cord. These nerves release chemicals which either cause the muscles of the digestive organs to squeeze with more force and increase the "push" of food and juice through the digestive tract, or they relax them. There is also a dense network of nerves inside the walls of the oesophagus, stomach, small intestine and colon. These nerves trigger contractions when food stretches

the walls of the intestine. They release many different substances that speed up or delay the movement of food and control when the digestive organs produce enzymes.

Normal bowel movements

How often is normal?

Most people do not pass a bowel motion just once a day. In Western parts of the world, like the UK, 'normal' can be anything from three times a day to once a week. In fact, the number of times you have a bowel movement can vary from day to day. The most common time to open your bowel is soon after you wake up or after a heavy meal.

What should it look like?

Doctors grade the form of the stool from 1 to 7 as follows.

1 Watery.

2 Mushy.

3 Soft.

4 Sausage- or banana-shaped.

5 Sausage- or banana-shaped but with cracks on the surface.

6 Lumpy and firm.

7 Separate hard lumps like peanuts or rabbit droppings.

The grades of 2 to 6 are said to be normal.

Producing gas

In the normal digestive system, the amount of gas passed through the anus varies from 500ml to 1500ml every day. Healthy people pass about 25ml to 100ml of gas about 14 times a day. Studies have shown that people with IBS pass the same amounts of gas as healthy people. It may be that with IBS, the muscles of the gut are very sensitive to the presence of gas which may lead to the upsetting symptoms of belching or burping, bloating, loud stomach rumbles and flatulence or farting.

There are different gases in different parts of the gut. The stomach and upper gut has oxygen, nitrogen and carbon dioxide. Oxygen and nitrogen come from air that is swallowed. Carbon dioxide is produced in the stomach. The colon contains hydrogen, methane and carbon dioxide. This gas is produced by bacteria in the colon which ferment the waste food products.

Diet and the digestive system

General advice about diet

The human body needs a balanced diet to work well. If you have the sort of IBS where your symptoms are related to the food you eat, do not cut out so much food that your diet becomes unbalanced. There are no hard and fast rules about diet but general good advice is to:

- eat meals at regular times;

- eat a wide variety of foods;

- balance the food you eat with physical activity; and

- aim for a 'healthy' weight.

The Balance of Good Health

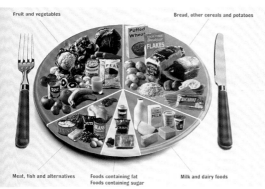

Reproduced with permission of Health Education Authority

The official guidelines for improving the average diet in the whole population of the United Kingdom are for people to:

- eat more, and a wider variety of, fruits and vegetables;

- eat less fat - especially saturated fat;

- eat more carbohydrate;

- eat more fibre;

- eat less salt; and

- drink alcohol in moderation.

This information is taken from the United Kingdom COMA (Committee on Medical Aspects of Food and Nutrition Policy) report.

There has been a great deal of research into the effect food can have on people with IBS. A lot of the research involves putting people on special diets where they are not allowed to eat certain food. These are known as exclusion diets. The food they are allowed to eat is very bland and is known not to upset the digestive system. If this diet stops the symptoms of IBS, foods are added back to the diet one item at a time. By keeping a careful record of people's symptoms on these diets, researchers have found that, in some people with IBS, certain types of food lead to symptoms.

The most common foods which lead to symptoms are listed in order below.

- Dairy products (milk, cheese and butter).

- Chocolate.

- Eggs.

- Wheat products.

- Nuts.

- Tea and coffee.

- Citrus fruits.

- Potatoes.

However, only a small number of people with IBS will have a reaction to food.

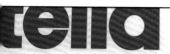

HAZELNUT CHOCOLATE SPREAD

INGREDIENTS: SUGAR,
VEGETABLE OILS, HAZELNUTS (13%),
FAT REDUCED COCOA POWDER,
LACTOSE, SKIMMED MILK POWDER (5%),
MILK PROTEINS, EMULSIFIER
(SOY LECITHIN), FLAVOURINGS.

400 g ℮

BEST BEFORE: SEE...

Nutrition:
100 g
27 kJ
3 kcal
6.5 g
57 g
31 g

Lactose intolerance

Lactose is a type of sugar which is found in milk and many processed foods (see page 37). There is a condition called lactose intolerance which has very similar symptoms to IBS. Lactose intolerance means your body cannot digest lactose. To digest lactose, the body has to produce an enzyme called lactase.

Lactase is normally produced by cells in the small intestine. Lactase breaks down milk sugar (lactose) into simpler forms that can then be absorbed into the bloodstream. If there is not enough lactase, milk sugar will reach the colon where it is broken down by bacteria to give 'short-chain fatty acids', carbon dioxide and hydrogen. This leads to:

● nausea;

● cramps;

● bloating;

● wind; and

● diarrhoea.

Symptoms begin about 30 minutes to two hours after eating or drinking foods containing lactose. How severe the symptoms are depends on the amount of lactose a person can tolerate.

25

In some studies up to one in five people with IBS who go to hospital clinics have been found to have lactose intolerance. There are simple tests which show whether you do not have enough lactase (in other words, whether you are lactase deficient).

Lactose intolerance tends to increase as people become adults, this is because less of the enzyme, lactase, is produced in the gut. Lactose intolerance affects certain population groups more than others. Nearly 100% of people from South East Asia have some lactose intolerance but less than 5% of people living in North-Western Europe are lactose intolerant.

There are many people with lactase deficiency who have no problems with milk products, and others with normal lactase who cannot tolerate milk products. **For people who have lactose intolerance and who cannot tolerate milk or milk products, it may be helpful to cut out food that contains lactose. If you think lactose intolerance may be a problem for you, please read the diet section in Chapter 4.** However, it is very rare that people need to avoid lactose totally.

Fibre in your diet

Fibre is important in everyone's diet. It is found in foods such as whole-grain cereals and breads, fruit and vegetables. There are different types of fibre and it is important to eat a variety of foods that are naturally high in fibre because these foods also supply vitamins, minerals and other nutrients. Fruit and vegetables contain substances such as 'bioflavinoids' which are thought to give us protection against cancer.

Most GPs ask their patients with IBS to eat more fibre because fibre does help relieve constipation. In Western parts of the world our diet tends to be low in fibre. Some studies have been done to look at what happens to people with IBS when they start to eat more bran fibre. These studies show that bran does not help relieve the symptoms of IBS for people with diarrhoea and it can make some symptoms worse. Remember that bran is only one of many sources of fibre.

If you have IBS with constipation, you are more likely to find that fibre helps you. A quick and easy way to eat more fibre is to sprinkle pure bran onto your cereal.

Adding more fibre to your diet may make problems worse for a short time as your gut gets used to the change. You should add more fibre to your diet slowly over several days. Adding more fibre to your diet may make you pass more wind. If you think you have a problem with fibre, it may be worth trying different types of fibre to see what product suits you best. You can find wholemeal products in health-food shops, look for the ones that are not wheat or bran based.

Things to remember

- We do not know what causes IBS.

- Tests show that people with IBS have nothing physically wrong with them.

- People with IBS have bowels that are sensitive and do not work properly.

- A healthy diet is important for the bowel to work properly.

Chapter 3
Medical tests

Introduction

Most people with IBS will not need any tests. It is possible to diagnose IBS without putting you through a lot of tests.

A diagnosis of IBS is based on your symptoms.

IBS is very common and if you have the following types of problems it is very unlikely that there is anything else wrong with you:

● symptoms which come and go;

● a pain in the abdomen which eases when you open your bowels; or

● a pain in the abdomen together with constipation or diarrhoea;

as well as any of the following symptoms:

● a change in the number of times you open your bowels;

● a change in the form of your stool - hard or loose;

● having to strain to open your bowels;

● feeling you have to open your bowels urgently;

● feeling you have not emptied your bowel fully;

● passing mucus (slime); or

● a bloated or swollen abdomen.

If you need to see a doctor or nurse, they will ask you about what you eat and about what medicines you are taking. They may also want to know about your lifestyle, work and any major stressful events in your life. It might help you to make a few notes to take with you when you see your doctor or nurse.

More serious problems

You may need more tests if you:

- are passing blood with your faeces;

- are losing weight;

- are waking up at night with pain or diarrhoea; or

- are over 40 when you first notice changes in your bowel movements.

If your main complaint is diarrhoea, you will need to give your GP a sample of your faeces to make sure you do not have an infection.

Most cases of bleeding from the rectum are not serious and are often due to damage to the lining of the bowel or rectum. If you have been straining to open your bowels to pass a hard stool, you may damage the lining of the bowel and it may bleed. If this is what has happened, the blood will be bright red (like a nosebleed). Or, the bleeding may mean that you have haemorrhoids (piles). **It is important for your doctor to confirm that the bleeding is not a sign of something more serious.** If you bleed from your rectum you should not ignore it, as it may be a symptom of a bowel disease or cancer.

If you have symptoms which you or your doctor think may be caused by something more serious, your GP should refer you to a gastroenterologist at the hospital. Your doctor will want to make sure you do not have bowel cancer or other gut disorders. The tests for this are as follows.

- Faecal occult blood test - this is where a sample of your faeces is tested to see if there is any blood in it.

- Blood tests.

- An examination of the inside of your rectum and colon by a special X-ray or by **sigmoidoscopy** or **colonoscopy**. This will be done by a specialist at the hospital.

Investigations
Barium X-ray

Barium is mixed into a liquid which shows up on X-rays. It is used when taking X-rays of the intestine because it will show up internal organs which don't normally show up on X-rays. It can be given orally (by mouth) or through the anus (an enema) depending on which part of your body is to be examined. If it is put into your body as an enema it may give you a strong urge to go to the toilet - but you will be asked to hold on until the examination is finished.

During a barium enema X-ray, you will be asked to move into different positions so that the barium will move up your colon from your rectum and coat the walls of your rectum and colon.

After taking barium your faeces will look chalky for one or two days. Tell your doctor if your faeces do not return to normal within a week, and you start to feel constipated.

A **double-contrast** study is when air is inserted with the barium to 'puff' up your colon and make any abnormalities much clearer to spot. Some people find this a little uncomfortable and it can cause cramping sensations or colicky pains similar to those of IBS.

Colonoscopy and sigmoidoscopy

A special tube is passed into your colon through your anus. The tube has a light in it and allows the doctor to look at your rectum and colon. The doctor can take samples (biopsies) from the lining of your colon and rectum during the test.

Medical tests

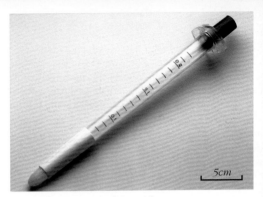

A rigid sigmoidoscope

A rigid **sigmoidoscope** is a short plastic tube which is inserted through your anus to look at your rectum and lower sigmoid colon. A **flexible sigmoidoscope** is longer and is used to look at the left side of the colon and can pass pictures on to a television screen. A **colonoscope** is used to look at the whole of the colon.

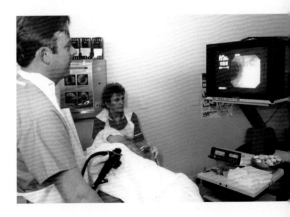

Your bowel will need to be prepared before a colonoscopy so that your colon is empty and clean before the examination. You will need to follow the instructions your hospital gives you very carefully. For two to three days before the examination you have to stop eating and can only drink clear fluids. You will also have to take a special medicine to clear out the faeces from your bowel. You will be offered sedation before the colonoscopy to make you sleepy and relaxed.

For a flexible sigmoidoscopy you will usually be given an enema about half an hour before the test. You will not need a special diet or medicine to clear your bowels. A rigid sigmoidoscopy can be performed without any preparation and is often done in the outpatient clinic.

If all the test results come out clear, you can feel reassured that you have IBS and nothing more serious. **Remember**, if your symptoms change from your normal pattern of IBS, you should tell your doctor.

'I felt better once I'd had some tests. Once I'd had them, I felt that I coped with it better, you know, I can laugh about it.'

Things to remember

● Most people with IBS do not need medical tests.

● If you are passing blood with your faeces, losing weight or being woken at night by pain, then you do need medical tests.

Chapter 4
What you can do to help yourself

This chapter looks at what **you** can do to help control your IBS.

Take control over your diet

We all know that certain food can upset our stomach and that food can upset people in different ways. There are many theories about how what we eat could be linked to IBS, but there is very little scientific evidence to base these theories on. Reactions to food depend on the person. True allergy to food is very rare, but many people are intolerant to certain foods. Many people complain of indigestion after eating certain foods (for example, celery, onions, garlic and cucumber) and tend to avoid them.

Modern diet

Some people think that our modern diet may cause IBS. There have been major changes in people's eating habits in the past 50 years.

- We eat less starchy food such as bread, oatmeal and potatoes.

- We eat more refined sugars and fats.

  Meals are often hurried or missed because of our hectic lifestyles.

- There has been a dramatic increase in the use of chemical food additives.

Diet is the most important change we can make to the environment of our digestive tract. These days, many people recognise the importance of a healthy diet because they have found that a healthy diet makes them feel better. There are more and more health-food shops and people are generally more aware of what they are eating. A healthy diet means eating plenty of fresh fruit and vegetables and eating foods which are low in fat and salt, and high in fibre.

'If I'm in pain one day, I'll go onto the high-fibre cereals and it does ease and help me.'

Food intolerance

People with IBS often find that certain foods bring on symptoms. The most common foods that people find cause problems are dairy products and wheat products. One way of finding out if food is causing IBS is to remove that food from your diet. Research has found that exclusion diets can get rid of the symptoms of IBS in some people. There is a big debate in the medical profession about the use of exclusion diets, as there is a worry that they may lead to some people becoming malnourished and ill.

Exclusion diets are hard going. You should not start such a diet on your own, because these diets are complicated and could be harmful if they are not done properly. Someone who is qualified, such as a dietitian, should supervise the diet. Exclusion diets are made up of foods which are known not to cause bad reactions. You have to stick to the diet strictly for at least two weeks for it to work. If your symptoms have gone by the end of the two weeks, you can start to add food back to your diet, one item at a time. You should be able to find out which food causes your symptoms. If your symptoms have not gone by the end of two weeks, you do not have food intolerance. If you want to try this strict diet, you should talk to your doctor or a qualified dietitian.

You may already know which types of food trigger your symptoms. If your IBS symptoms are not too severe, you can work out for yourself if certain food causes problems. Remember to cut out one type of food at a time. Use a food diary to help you remember which food you have eaten in the 24 hours before a bad attack.

'Milk seems to upset me quite a lot, and I love milk.'

Examples of food most likely to cause IBS symptoms

The symptoms you have may be caused by lactose intolerance. You can test this simply by cutting out dairy products. If you have lactose intolerance your symptoms will stop when you do this.

Dairy products are:

- milk;
- cream;
- butter;
- ice cream;
- cheese; and
- cottage cheese.

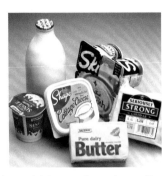

Yoghurt is a dairy product which contains only small amounts of lactose. The bacteria used to make yoghurt from milk turn some of the lactose into lactic acid. If you have lactose intolerance, you may be able to eat yoghurt without getting IBS symptoms.

Processed foods contain added lactose. You should check the list of ingredients.

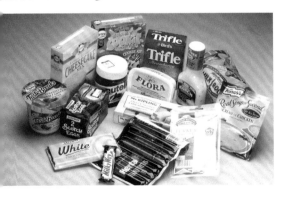

Examples of processed foods are:

- bread and other baked foods;
- processed breakfast cereals;
- instant mashed potatoes, soups, and breakfast drinks;
- margarine;
- lunch meats (other than kosher);
- salad dressings;
- sweets and other snacks; and
- mixes for pancakes and biscuits.

Some food which is labelled as 'non-dairy', such as powdered coffee whitener and whipped toppings, may also include ingredients that come from milk and contain lactose.

You may find that you do not need to cut out dairy products completely. Just cutting down on milk might be enough to prevent your symptoms. Your body should be able to digest small amounts of lactose without causing problems. It may help to eat other food at the same time as you eat or drink a dairy product.

If you have lactose intolerance and you cut down on food containing lactose, your symptoms will completely clear.

Remember that dairy products are an important source of calcium, which is needed all through your life to grow, maintain and repair bones.

Everyone needs calcium, especially growing children and women who have been through the menopause to prevent osteoporosis (thin bones). Cheese and yoghurt are good sources of calcium and you may be able to eat these even if you cannot tolerate milk.

What you can do to help yourself

Other good sources of calcium are:

  fish with soft bones which you can eat (such as salmon and sardines); and

  calcium-enriched soya milk which you can get from supermarkets and health-food shops.

If you avoid all these foods, you can get general advice on calcium supplements from health-food shops. If you are very concerned, a dietitian will be able to check your diet and tell you whether you need a calcium supplement.

Wheat products

Some people with IBS have problems eating wheat products. This is usually because wheat products are quite stodgy.

Examples of wheat products are:

- bread;

- pastry; and

- breakfast cereals that are wheat based (oat-based cereals should not cause a problem).

Artificial sweeteners and some types of sugar have been found to lead to symptoms of IBS, for example:

- sorbitol; and

- fructose.

Sorbitol is actually a laxative and causes diarrhoea even in people who do not have digestive problems.

Drinks

People have suggested that coffee and alcohol can cause problems because they may dehydrate you (remove water from your system). If there is not enough fluid in your digestive system, you can have problems digesting food and your constipation will be worse.

Fruit and vegetables

People with IBS often say they have problems after eating fruit and vegetables. Good nutritional advice is to eat at least five portions of fruit or vegetables a day. A glass of pure fruit juice counts as one portion of fruit. Some people who have IBS with diarrhoea have problems if they eat this amount of fruit and vegetables. You need to find out what suits you. People with constipation should find their symptoms improve when they eat more fruit and vegetables.

Food allergies

It is very unlikely that your IBS is due to a food allergy. Many people think they are allergic to certain food because it causes them discomfort. This is likely to be an intolerance to the food, which can cause distressing symptoms but is not dangerous. In medicine, an allergic reaction is when the immune system reacts with something to cause symptoms such as rashes, facial swelling or difficulty in breathing. These are serious and life threatening, for example a peanut or strawberry allergy. Only a very small number of people have true food allergies.

Tests for allergies and intolerance

A food challenge is when you are given a small amount of a food to eat that you think may cause a reaction. The food can be hidden in a capsule so that you don't know what you have eaten.

Skin prick tests and blood tests are sometimes used to see if you are allergic to items of food. These tests are not reliable because they often show a positive reaction to foods which do not cause problems and may not show up true allergies..

Gas problems

As mentioned earlier, people with IBS often report problems with wind. They have belching or burping, a bloated feeling, loud stomach rumbles and flatulence or farting. These symptoms can all be very distressing.

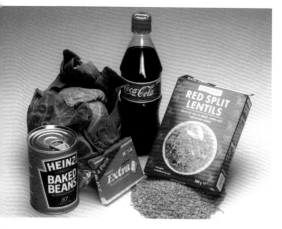

Certain foods produce a lot of gas. For example:

- baked beans and other beans;

- cabbage and brussel sprouts;

- lentils;

- apples and apple juice; and

- grapes.

To reduce the amount of gas in the stomach do not:

- drink fizzy drinks;

- chew chewing gum; or

- eat your food quickly.

I love carbonated water, I find if I put just a drop of lime juice in, it takes the fizz out.'

Gut fermentation

People are beginning to wonder if the type and amount of bacteria in the gut are important. There are more than 400 types of bacteria in the human gut and researchers do not yet know how important they are for our health. We need bacteria in the colon to ferment food products. Some people believe this process may not be working properly in people with IBS. They suggest that something, perhaps infection or antibiotics, has changed the types of bacteria in the gut. If the normal gut bacteria are not there, then it is possible for other micro-organisms such as yeasts to take their place. Yeasts ferment food in a different way to normal gut bacteria and it is suggested this difference can cause the symptoms of IBS in some people. There is not yet enough research evidence to know if this is a true cause of IBS.

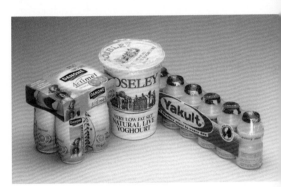

Probiotics are foods which contain live bacteria such as *Lactobacillus acidophilus* and *Bifobacterium bifidium* which are said to be beneficial to health. Live bacteria are found in live yoghurts such as Bio yoghurts and fermented milk drinks.

Prebiotics are substances you can eat that are food for certain friendly bacteria in the colon and stimulate their growth. You can buy prebiotics in health-food shops. Examples of prebiotics are whey protein and fructo-oligosaccharides (FOS).

Medical research has not yet shown that probiotics and prebiotics help people with IBS, but there is no research to prove they do not work and many people have found them helpful.

'I started taking Yakult. I can't say I'm better but I'm not as uncomfortable, I seem to cope better.'

Your diet

If you think your IBS may be caused by what you eat, you can try to change your diet. It is easy to become obsessed by food when you have IBS and if you are not careful, you can fall into the trap of cutting out a lot of food when you don't need to. If you have stopped eating one type of food because you think it causes you problems, it is worth trying it again at a later date. You do have to be a detective about your diet, because everyone's reaction to food is so different. What works for one person may make someone else feel worse. Remember that keeping to a regular eating pattern will help.

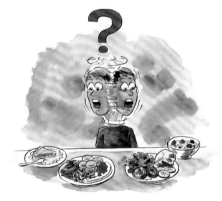

Some foods help some people . . .

'Yakult seemed to help for a while, to soothe it.'

'If I don't eat fruit, I find I have problems.'

'I eat a banana each morning, I don't have to rush t the toilet like I used to.'

'I eat a lot of green vegetables in a stir fry. I find when I eat stir fry, I eat a lot slower, I chew.'

'I've found that porridge helps me.'

'If I'm feeling really bad, I'll just have some soup, it relieves it a bit.'

'When I'm bad, I have white boiled rice and lumps o chicken in sauce.'

. . . but make others worse

'High fibre caused diarrhoea that I couldn't control. was walking around using nappies because I just couldn't control it after Bran Flakes.'

'I can't touch bananas, they just go right through me.'

'Oranges affect me quite badly, fresh oranges.'

'Cherry tomatoes, I had them in a sandwich and on Sunday morning I was absolutely creased with wind rushing to the loo, faecal soiling.'

'If I eat sprouts, ooh I get wind pains.'

'I've cut out things with bits in, like granary bread and crunchy peanut butter. That does alleviate it a bit, I wondered if the bits were aggravating it.'

'I think keeping off the fatty foods has helped in the actual need to go to the toilet.'

'I think spicy food's another thing that can trigger it off. Like curries and things.'

'If I go to a do and I eat a lot of sausage rolls and pastries, next day I will have stomach ache.'

44

Ways of eating

Some people have found that the way they eat can lead to symptoms of IBS. Eating quickly and gulping air can lead to problems.

It's in the pattern of eating more than what I actually eat. If I rush food, that doesn't help and if I eat a large meal rather than smaller meals throughout the day, that doesn't help.'

'If I pig out, that's when I have bloating.'

Exercise

We know that as well as keeping the body fit, exercise leads to a sense of well-being. Exercise may be especially helpful to people with IBS because:

- being active helps with constipation problems;

- exercise makes you feel better about yourself;

- it is easier to relax after exercise;

- exercise helps you to keep a healthy body weight; and

  exercise reduces your appetite.

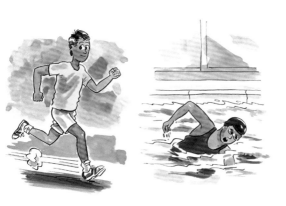

Here are some tips on exercise

- Try a kind of exercise which uses most of the large muscles of the body, for example, walking, running or swimming.

- Introduce exercise slowly in both the amount of effort and time you put into it. You should increase the amount of exercise you do in small stages over several weeks.

- The exercise should make you sweat and feel out of breath for some part of the time, but you should still be able to talk during the exercise.

- You should exercise for at least 20 minutes, three times a week.

'It's hard to do stomach exercises when you're really bloated and it is hurting you, but doing sit ups and stomach exercises gets it moving, gets it working.'

How to deal with stress

Relaxation

Learning how to relax may be helpful to people with IBS for two reasons:

- relaxing is a way you can manage and reduce stress; and

- relaxing may be a way you can relieve pain.

Relaxation may work by breaking the vicious circle:

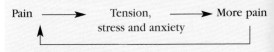

Pain ⟶ Tension, stress and anxiety ⟶ More pain

There are several ways of teaching yourself to relax. Relaxation is something you can practice and get better at. It is also possible to be taught how to relax in a class or by a therapist. Many women are taught relaxation techniques during ante-natal classes when they are pregnant.

Stress

Stress is often said to lead to IBS. Most people with IBS say they can link a stressful event to their symptoms. Sometimes stress can be a good thing, we need a certain amount of stress to make us act and think about what we are doing. But stress can become harmful if we can't cope or don't know how to cope with what is causing the stress. Some people may become stressed more easily than others. These are people who have:

- poor health;

- no work;

- financial worries;

- a complicated life and work style;

- a lack of effective ways of coping with difficult situations;

- emotional problems;

- bad previous experiences; or

- low self confidence.

If you think your IBS is linked to stress, there may be ways to manage stress better. You may need to make changes in your:

- lifestyle and working environment; and

- behaviour, and in the way you use your body.

Sometimes it is not possible to deal with the cause of the stress because it is outside your control. However, there are things you can do to reduce the effects of stress.

- Try to exercise for at least 20 minutes, three times a week. Exercise is also good for IBS as it prevents constipation. You can join an exercise class or take a brisk walk in the evening.

- Improve the way you stand and sit.

47

- Develop healthy eating habits (see page 23).

- Stop smoking and drinking alcohol or at least try to reduce the amount you smoke or drink.

- Talk to others, such as friends or family, who might be supportive.

- Listen to music and read books.

- Take up relaxing hobbies - such as fishing.

Learning how to relax your body can help to ease stress. Relaxation may also help relieve pain. There are simple ways to relax at work during the day.

- Short, frequent breaks (for five minutes every hour) are more relaxing than fewer, longer breaks.

- Small physical exercises are helpful for people who use computers, for example, tensing and relaxing muscles in your legs and arms.

- Take a few deep breaths and breathe out slowly to try to stop an immediate stress reaction or panic attack.

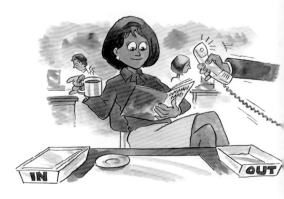

There are three parts to the most successful relaxation techniques.

1. You should focus on a word or action which you keep repeating.

2. You should ignore passing thoughts.

3. You should relax your muscles.

Relaxation therapy has been shown to be of use in many situations and should be helpful to most people with IBS. Try to spend half an hour a day relaxing in a place where you won't be disturbed. Quiet soothing music can help. There are many relaxation tapes on the market.

I've had a lot of those tapes and one with colours, and one with dreams, walking by the river and things like that, so ... you just try them really, but they help with calming you down.'

Progressive relaxation training

The following section is an example of a common technique which is taught in relaxation classes. This technique teaches you to tense up and release groups of muscles around your body. The aim is to make your muscles relax. A firm contraction leads to a deep relaxation. You need to become aware of the feelings you get in your body when you tense and release muscles. There are 16 muscle groups to tense and release and it takes 20 to 30 minutes to go through it all.

1. Make a fist with your right hand without using your upper arm. *Then relax and think about how your muscles feel.*

2. Push your right elbow down against the arm of the chair while your hand is relaxed. *Then relax and think about how your muscles feel.*

3. Make a fist with your left hand without using your upper arm. *Then relax and think about how your muscles feel.*

4 Push your left elbow down against the arm of the chair while your hand is relaxed. *Then relax and think about how your muscles feel.*

5 Raise your eyebrows. *Then relax and think about how your muscles feel.*

6 Screw up your eyes and wrinkle your nose. *Then relax and think about how your muscles feel.*

7 Clench your teeth and pull back the corners of your mouth. *Then relax and think about how your muscles feel.*

8 Pull your chin down and press your head back against a support, for example the back of your chair, tense your neck muscles. *Then relax and think about how your muscles feel.*

9 Draw your shoulders back. *Then relax and think about how your muscles feel.*

10 Tighten your abdominal muscles (make your stomach hard). *Then relax and think about how your muscles feel.*

11 Tense the thigh of your right leg by contracting the muscles which go to your knee. *Then relax and think about how your muscles feel.*

12 Point your right foot down. *Then relax and think about how your muscles feel.*

13 Pull your right foot up towards your face. *Then relax and think about how your muscles feel.*

14 Tense the thigh of your left leg by contracting the muscles which go to your knee. *Then relax and think about how your muscles feel.*

15 Point your left foot down. *Then relax and think about how your muscles feel.*

16 Pull your left foot up towards your face. *Then relax and think about how your muscles feel.*

You should practise this twice a day for 15 to 20 minutes. When you feel you have practised this well and are able to relax fully, you can cut down to four items.

1. Work both of your arms together.

2. Work your face and head together.

3. Work your neck and body together.

4. Work both legs together.

Breathing and relaxation

You can do breathing exercises anywhere. Calm breathing has a slow rate and is done with the abdominal muscles relaxed. Stressful breathing is faster, involves the rib muscles and makes the shoulders tense.

Relax your jaw to help you to breathe slowly.

Let your lower jaw drop slightly, as if you were starting a small yawn. Keep your tongue still and resting in the bottom of your mouth. Let your lips go soft. Breathe slowly and in a three-beat pattern of breathe in, breathe out and rest. Stop forming words, don't even think about words.'

Another way to breathe slowly:

Breathe in slowly and deeply. As you breathe out slowly, feel yourself starting to relax. Feel the tension leaving you. Now breathe in and out slowly and regularly at a comfortable rate.

Focus on your breathing. As you breathe in and as you breathe out, say to yourself, "One, two, three." Or each time you breathe out, repeat a focus word like "peace" or "relax" or "I feel calm and relaxed".'

A slightly different way:

Listen to your breathing. Imagine your tensions being breathed out, a little at a time with each breath out. Imagine that each time you breathe in, you are

breathing in peace a little at a time. Breathe out
tension, breathe in peace, gently breathing, feeling
peace flowing through your body.'

Things to remember

You can control your IBS by yourself by:

● changing your diet;

● taking more exercise; and

● taking action to reduce stress.

Chapter 5
More ways to manage your IBS

This chapter will tell you about types of treatment you can try which do not involve going to the doctor.

Complementary therapy

Complementary therapies aim to treat 'the whole person'. People with IBS are sometimes so fed up with the lack of help they get from usual medical treatment that they want to try alternative therapies as well to see if a different approach will work for them. This can be expensive, but many people find complementary therapies very helpful. Products in health-food shops or those which you can buy over the counter in a pharmacy can be fairly cheap, but it gets more expensive if you pay for a therapist to give you treatment. A few doctors' practices offer complementary or alternative therapies to their patients. Many complementary therapies have not been tested in the way that medicines and treatments are tested in conventional medicine. Western medicine cannot explain how alternative treatments work.

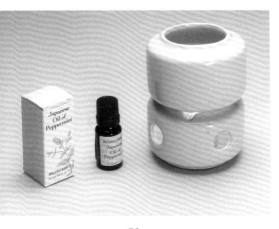

Does complementary therapy work for IBS?

Aromatherapy and abdominal massage

Aromatherapy uses essential oils which have been extracted from plants. There are written records about the use of aromatic oils which go back to the time of the ancient Greeks and the Egyptians, but aromatherapy has only recently become popular as a therapy in the United Kingdom. The oils contain compounds which aromatherapists believe have various healing properties. Peppermint oils are said to help people with digestive problems. Certain types of oils are said to help with the different symptoms of IBS. The oils are said to increase the well-being of the mind and the body.

The following table shows you which symptoms of IBS aromatherapists suggest the different oils may help with.

Oil	Pain	Diarrhoea	Constipation	Bloating and wind
Basil	Yes			Yes
Bergamot	Yes			Yes
Black pepper	Yes	Yes	Yes	Yes
Camomile			Yes	Yes
Clary sage				Yes
Fennel			Yes	Yes
Ginger		Yes		Yes
Juniper	Yes			Yes
Lavender		Yes		Yes
Peppermint		Yes		Yes
Rosemary	Yes	Yes		Yes

The oils can be taken into the body through the nose, skin, rectum or vagina. Rubbing the oils into the skin by massage is a common form of therapy. The oils are absorbed both through the skin and by breathing in the vapours.

Massage is an important part of the therapy because it is relaxing and eases physical and mental stress.

Aromatherapy is something you can try for yourself. There are many aromatherapy products available and it is well worth trying the oils yourself to see if certain ones help you. You can use the oils in many ways.

- They can be massaged onto the skin of your abdomen.

- You can put them into your bath.

- You can put a few drops on a handkerchief and breathe in deeply.

- You can heat the oil and breathe in the fumes by putting a few drops into a small bowl of water placed over a candle inside an essential oil burner.

You can use up to four oils at a time - the nose can only cope with three to four different smells. Choose the oils you like the smell of and use a few drops of each.

Relaxing oils include:

- camomile;

- juniper;

- lavender;

- marjoram;

- sandalwood; and

- ylang ylang.

Invigorating oils include:

● eucalyptus;

● bergamot;

● lemon;

● peppermint; and

● rosemary.

To deal with stress, try mixing lavender, geranium and sandalwood.

Some research has been done on aromatherapy and it is said to help people with IBS, particularly people with symptoms of pain. You may find it helpful to get treatment from an aromatherapist who will be able to give you an aromatherapy massage as well as help you to find a mix of oils to help with your IBS symptoms. Different oils help people in different ways.

Massage is relaxing and it eases physical and mental stress.

Health-food shops and many major stores sell aromatherapy oils, and it is worth experimenting with different types to find out what suits you. The oils themselves may cause side effects and if you are pregnant, you should not use some oils, including basil, hyssop, sage and thyme. Using large amounts of aromatherapy oils may cause problems. Never swallow essential oils or use them undiluted on the skin.

Aromatherapy is a new type of complementary treatment. There are no laws in the United Kingdom about how much training an aromatherapist should have. European laws say that the only medical claims a therapist can make are that the therapy reduces stress.

Acupuncture
Acupuncture is a traditional Chinese medicine. It is said to help with the symptoms of some medical conditions and may help the body to heal itself. It is known to increase the body's natural painkillers and has been shown to be of some help to people with

hronic pain. Fine needles are inserted through the
kin. The number of needles varies but may be only
wo or three. The average number of visits for
reatment is about five.

ome GPs will refer patients to a private acupuncture
linic, but a few acupuncture clinics are available on
he NHS. There are many people in the UK who are
ualified to practise acupuncture. There is some
esearch which shows acupuncture might be helpful
o people whose IBS causes bloating.

eflexology

eflexology is a treatment where pressure is applied
o the feet or hands to promote health and well-being.
he therapist will massage the feet or hands in a
pecial way. It is said to work because of reflexes or
ones which run through the body and end in the feet
r hands. All the systems and organs of the body are
aid to be represented by an area on the surface of the
oot or hand. The therapist applies gentle pressure to
he matching area on the foot or hand to treat any
roblem in that part of the body.

nyone can learn how to do reflexology and become
 reflexologist. There are many training courses in the
K.

eflexology has been used as a therapy in India and
hina for thousands of years. There is some research
vidence that it can help to reduce pain and help
eople to relax deeply, but no specific research has
een done to study the use of reflexology for people
ith IBS. Reflexology may help people who have IBS
ymptoms they can relate to stress.

olonic irrigation

olonic irrigation involves passing a tube into the
ectum and putting a large volume of water into the
owel. Colonic irrigation is not recommended by
edical specialists as it has no known health benefits,
nd it does have serious dangers as it can lead to
amage and tearing of the colon.

Yoga

Yoga exercises are designed to improve muscle tone, flexibility, and circulation as well as improving the well-being of the mind. Yoga comes from an Eastern tradition where health is seen as a state of balance between the body, mind and spirit. Doing yoga exercises as a daily routine has been shown to reduce physical tension. Research has shown that yoga may help to speed up recovery from stressful situations, relieve insomnia (when you can't sleep at night), and improve concentration and energy.

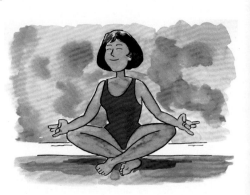

At yoga classes, you learn a total body relaxation technique followed by meditation, a way to quiet the mind so that it rests from daily stresses. Regular meditation practice can teach you how to relax whenever you need to.

Transcendental meditation

Transcendental meditation is a simple way to become deeply relaxed. It is a very old tradition that started in India thousands of years ago and is now practised by millions of people all over the world. You are supposed to practise it for 20 minutes in the morning and evening using a special word called a 'mantra'. Many doctors and nurses recommend it to their patients. Research has shown that transcendental meditation can lower the blood pressure and certain stress-related chemicals in the body.

'I suppose when you look at the cost of the pills that they're pushing, it would be better to spend it on transcendental meditation. Cos it's only 20 minutes, I do mine once in a morning and once on a night, and I find it very beneficial.'

You will have to pay to go on a course of classes to learn the technique of transcendental meditation. There is an address at the end of the book if you want more information.

'I've done visual meditation. I try and calm myself down and then visualise the medicine bottle and it's the one that's going to cure me. And it's there, imaginary, IBS down, go, gone. So send it off.'

Talking to others

You can feel very alone when you have IBS. It helps if you have someone sympathetic who will work with you to find out the best way to manage your IBS. Most of you will find you have a friend, work colleague or relative who also has IBS. It might help to talk to them.

Many doctors' practices have a counsellor. This is someone who is trained to listen carefully to people's problems and who can offer general advice about coping with stress and anxiety. There is research to show that people find counselling helpful but there is no research to show that it is of special help to people with IBS.

'Counsellors are trained to listen and sometimes, because somebody's actually listened to what you're thinking about, it makes a world of a difference.'

Self-help groups can provide a lot of support. There is a national support group for people with IBS called the IBS Network (the address and phone number are at the end of this guide).

A national group will send you newsletters and keep you up to date with new treatments for IBS.

Herbal treatments and health-food shops

Chinese herbal medicine is one treatment that has been proved to work for IBS. Chinese herbal medicine has been used for many centuries in China to treat bowel disorders. The treatment used has to be tailored to the person by someone who practises Chinese medicine. Research has shown that symptoms of IBS can be improved a lot by taking Chinese herbal medicine.

Many people with IBS buy remedies from health-food shops. There is a wide range of products you can try such as:

- aloe vera (in many forms);

- oil of peppermint;

- essential oils for aromatherapy;

- probiotic products containing live bacteria (see page 42);

- soya milk;

- herbal teas; and

- bran (wheat and oat bran).

People with IBS have very different stories about what happens to them when they take treatments such as aloe vera or herbal remedies.

'I ordered aloe vera because there'd been an article in the paper how good it was for stomach complaints and I really thought that was it, this was gonna cure me. It did absolutely nothing. It's like £12 down the drain.'

'I took some peppermint tea, and that seemed to calm the pain down a bit.'

hewing root ginger is said to help with digestion. erb teas such as camomile, ginger and peppermint re also helpful.

'just tried something that was suggested two years go, and it's been quite helpful and that is Slippery lm. You can buy it in the tablet form and you can ix it like a paste, it's a very old-fashioned thing, but f a night time mix this powder, and it seems to uieten the digestive tract, the whole lot, it helps with e wind and everything.'

ver-the-counter treatments

is possible to buy medicines to treat IBS from a harmacy without a prescription.

eople who have had IBS for a long time, sometimes el that there is no cure that doctors can offer them. octors tend to treat the symptoms of IBS, because ere are medicines which will deal with pain, onstipation, diarrhoea and intestinal gas. In most ases, it is possible to buy a medicine that will help ou with your symptoms. Remember that these edicines do not cure IBS. Because there are so many ymptoms of IBS, there are many treatments and what ight work for one person, may not work for another.

' don't think many drugs actually work. You're just ontrolling the diarrhoea, it's not getting rid of the BS problem.'

'eppermint oil capsules are lovely. The wind, I was umbling like billy-o, it's horrible noises, but it helps.'

Some facts about medicines to help you choose the right one for your symptoms

Drugs for constipation

Do not use laxatives on a regular basis. The simplest treatment for constipation is to:

- eat more fibre;

- drink more fluid; and

- take more exercise. Exercise will help with constipation because using the large muscles of th body helps to move the contents of the colon. If you are not active, you are far more likely to be constipated.

If these steps do not work, there are several types of laxatives you can buy for IBS. They have different effects on the bowel.

Bulking agents are made from plant fibre or methylcellulose. They make the mass of faeces larger. They do this by absorbing water which also makes the faeces softer. A large mass of faeces will start the action of peristalsis (muscle movement of the bowel wall). It may take some days before there is any effect It is important to drink a lot when you are taking bulking agents to avoid blockages in the gut.

You should take bulking agents with a glass of water in the evening or morning - not just before you go to bed

Examples of bulking agents are:

- bran - Trifyba;

- ispaghula husk - Fybogel, Konsyl, Isogel and Regulan;

- sterculia - Normacol; and

- methylcellulose - Celevac.

Osmotic laxatives draw water into the bowel to make faeces easier to pass. It is important to drink a lot when you are taking these laxatives.

Examples of osmotic laxatives are:

lactulose - Duphalac, Lacitol, Lactugal, Regulose, Movicol.

People with IBS should not need to take stimulant laxatives. They increase muscle movement in the colon and can cause cramping pain. They take about six to 12 hours to work.

Examples of stimulant laxatives are:

senna - Manevac, Senakot.

Drugs for diarrhoea

There are drugs you can buy which help to slow down the action of the muscles of the bowel. These drugs are called **antimotility drugs**.

Examples of antimotility drugs are:

loperamide, Arret, Diasorb, Diocalm; and

kaoline and morphine - Enterosan, Opazimes.

If you sometimes get constipation and sometimes get diarrhoea, laxatives and drugs for constipation can sometimes make the symptoms worse.

Drugs for pain

Drugs can be used to relax the muscles of the gut. It is thought that these tightenings of the muscles or 'spasm' are the cause of the pain suffered by some people with IBS.

There are antispasmodic drugs you can buy which relax the muscle of the gut.

Examples of antispasmodic drugs are:

- merbeverine hydrochloride - Colofac;

- alverine citrate - Spasmonal, Alvercol; and

- peppermint oil - Colpermin, Mintec.

Wind

Charcoal is a non-prescription medicine that some people say works for wind.

'Charcoal tablets really helped with the embarrassing wind problem.'

The placebo effect

The placebo effect happens during trials of new drug or treatments. It is when someone's symptoms get better even though they are not taking the active drug. The treatment they are given is a dummy pill or therapy which looks the same as the real thing but has no active parts.

It is thought that some people get better when they have placebo treatment partly because of the interest the person giving the therapy has in their condition and in the attention they get. In fact, all treatments whether or not they have active parts have a psychological effect on the patient.

The placebo effect clearly shows the strong link between the brain and the body because in all research trials, many people do get better without active treatment.

If you have confidence in the treatment you are given the treatment is more likely to cure you. Many doctors think this is one of the reasons that many therapies work. There is often no known scientific reason why the therapy should work. People may feel better because someone has spent a lot of time talking to them about their symptoms. Of course, there may be something about the therapy that works on the body in a way that medicine is not yet able to measure.

Things to remember

- Complementary therapy can be helpful for people with IBS.

- Health-food shops are a source of IBS remedies.

- Over-the-counter medicines can help with symptoms of IBS.

Chapter 6
Medical treatments

What can you do if nothing seems to be helping?

This chapter will tell you about the medical treatments used to help people with IBS who have not been able to manage the condition on their own. About 95% of people with IBS should be able to manage their IBS using the simple methods in this guide. But there are a small number of people who have very bad symptoms which are not helped by any treatment. If none of the methods in this guide have helped, you might need to think about other therapies.

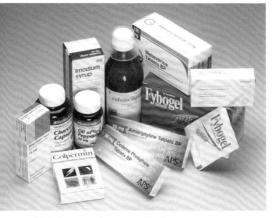

Drugs which have to be prescribed by a doctor

The following drug information is taken from the British National Formulary which is a guidebook doctors use when prescribing medicines.

Drugs for diarrhoea

Antimotility drugs slow down the action of the muscles of the bowel.

65

Examples of antimotility drugs are:

- loperamide - Imodium;

- co-phenotrope - Lomotil; and

- codeine phosphate.

Drugs for pain
Anticholinergics act on the nerve supply to the muscles of the gut. They have side effects which include a dry mouth and blurred vision.

Examples of anticholinergics are:

- dicyclomine hydrochloride - Merbentyl; and

- hyoscine butylbromide - Buscopan.

There are other antispasmodic drugs which relax the muscle of the gut but which do not have the side effects of anticholinergics, for example:

- mebeverine hydrochloride - Colofac.

Tricyclic antidepressant therapy
Recent research has found that low doses of antidepressant drugs may be helpful for some IBS symptoms. Tricyclic antidepressants have been shown to act on the muscles of the bowel and may be helpful to people with symptoms of pain. These drugs do sometimes have side effects including tiredness, dry mouth and not passing urine. These side effects usually wear off in a few days.

IBS may also be a feature of depression. People may not realise they are depressed. Depression does have an effect on the body and makes people feel pain more easily, the spasms and movements of the muscles in the gut are felt more sharply. Depression makes people feel tired and not want to exercise, and a lack of exercise causes constipation. Antidepressants may be helpful both to deal with depression and to ease the symptoms of pain.

xamples of antidepressants used for IBS:

Imipramine; and

Desipramine.

ecent studies show that some of the newer
ntidepressants such as Fluoxetine (Prozac) may also
elp people with irritable bowel syndrome.

sychotherapy

sychotherapy is a treatment where you are helped to
nderstand the physical effects emotional upsets and
tresses have on your body. These could be concerns
bout money, your family or your job. It is known that
sychological disturbances can cause bowel
roblems. If you are helped with problems of anxiety
nd depression, then it has been shown that your
owel symptoms can be improved as well. For
sychotherapy to work well, it seems to be very
mportant that you develop a good relationship with
he therapist. If you feel you need to see a
sychotherapist, your GP or hospital specialist may
efer you or you can contact a psychotherapist
rivately.

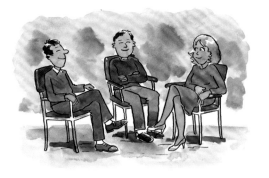

Behavioural therapy

Behavioural therapy is when you are taught how to understand and control your psychological or physical symptoms. It is possible to pay for sessions of group-therapy with other IBS sufferers. You will learn:

● how the bowel works;

● how to recognise what can trigger your IBS; and

● different ways of coping with IBS (such as relaxation, medication, diet, stress and anxiety management, and gut-directed hypnosis).

Being with a group can be very supportive.

Hypnotherapy

Hypnosis is said to be a way of gaining access to the unconscious mind. It is a skill that people can learn so that they can use their mind in a different way. A hypnotic trance is a state of focused attention. It is like when you are so absorbed in a book or film that you do not hear what someone says to you.

Hypnotherapists may have different ways of dealing with IBS. There are no strict controls over who can do hypnotherapy. If you decide to try hypnotherapy, it is important that you go to someone who has experience in gut-directed hypnotherapy. Go to a registered therapist who has been recommended by someone you trust.

Hypnotherapy can be used to help you relax and to overcome stress. Not everyone will benefit from hypnotherapy.

Gut-directed hypnotherapy is a way of aiming the treatment at the problems of IBS. This method has been shown to work for some patients with severe IBS. The gut can be affected by the mind, so hypnotherapists say they are teaching you skills to control your gut in a 'mind-over-matter' way. It is not a cure, but many people who have had gut-directed hypnotherapy find that their symptoms are much nproved, and they feel better in themselves and more ble to cope with life.

his is just one example of gut-directed ypnotherapy

● You will be told how the gut works and what might be going wrong with it.

● You will be given an hourly session of hypnotherapy once a week for three months.

The hypnotherapy will be aimed at the gut. You will be told to put your hand on your tummy and to feel warmth. You will then be told to relate this feeling to the relief of pain, spasm and bloating of IBS. You will also be asked to think up a picture of a river and to imagine that it is your gut. You will be told to change the way the river is flowing so that your bowels will work better. For example, if you are having problems with loose bowels, you will be asked to imagine that a fast-flowing river is changed to a slow, smoothly flowing one.

● You will be asked to do self-hypnosis at home by listening to a tape.

Things to remember

● A few people with IBS may benefit from medical help.

● Prescription drugs may give you side effects.

● Only a few people need professional psychological help.

Chapter 7
Summary
and sources of information

This chapter is a summary of what you can do to
cope with and manage your IBS. Remember, we do
not know how to cure IBS but we do know that
things improve when people take control and manage
their IBS instead of letting it manage them.

*'I think there must be something out there for
everybody that will help you manage it better. It's just
finding the right thing for the individual person isn't
it?'*

Coping plans

1. Be clear about what your symptoms are and which
   symptoms you find most troublesome. Check you
   have the symptoms listed on page 29.

2. Feel reassured that if you have IBS, there is nothing
   more serious going on.

3. Try to work out what triggers off your IBS.

4. Change your diet if you need to.

5. Think about what makes you feel stressed.

6. Do more exercise.

7. Learning how to relax properly may help.

8. You may find it helpful to find someone else with
   IBS and talk to them.

9. Consider whether complementary therapies might
   help you.

10. Work with your doctor, nurse or therapist to find a
    method to ease your symptoms.

General tips

1. Unless you already eat a high-fibre diet, slowly
   increase the amount of fibre you eat. Most people
   do need more fibre in their diet. Fibre will help

with constipation and may help with diarrhoea. If you suddenly start to eat large amounts of food with a high-fibre content you may get stomach pains and cramps as your body tries to fit in with the new diet. You will also pass more wind and fee bloated until your body learns to cope with the added fibre. This will take about two to three weeks. Some people with IBS cannot cope with a high-fibre diet as it makes their symptoms worse. You can only find this out by experience.

2 Drink more water. More water in your diet will help with constipation and diarrhoea. You should try to drink eight to ten glasses of water a day.

3 Develop good bowel habits.

● Do not take laxatives on a regular basis.

● When you have the urge to open your bowels, do not hold on, try to go as soon as you can.

● Do not strain when you are trying to open your bowels. If your motion does not come in a minute or so, get off the toilet and wait for the urge to come back.

● Do not hold on to wind.

4 Exercise more often. Using the muscles of your abdomen will help to move the contents of your bowel in a more regular way.

5 Try simple methods of pain relief - a hot-water bottle on your tummy should be soothing.

'I have a lie in the bath and keep topping it up.'

'I go to bed and stay there with a hot-water bottle.'

'I'll have a game of patience with my coffee and I find it does make me sit and take a bit more time before I'm rushing about.'

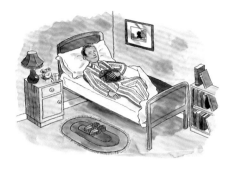

Detective work

You will need to find out what is happening to your body. Think about your symptoms.

What are they?

When do you get them?

Can you link them to anything that has happened in your life?

Could your IBS be linked to food?

Action

When your IBS feels as if it is out of your control, it may be helpful to keep a diary of your symptoms for about two weeks. You can record the time the attacks happened, how bad they were and whether you can link them to anything such as the food you have eaten, work problems or problems at home.

Medication

Work out which drugs will help with your symptoms. Try to find a drug to deal with the symptom which gives you the most trouble. There is no one drug which works for everyone with IBS.

'I tried all the medication. All the sorts of things I've had, I've exchanged one problem for something else, more stomach ache or headaches.'

'If I'm going somewhere special and I feel gripey, I take a couple of loperamide tablets, those always work.'

Problems with sex

Many men and women with severe symptoms of IBS say they have problems with sex. The main problem people have is a reduction in sex drive. People who have IBS with constipation are more likely to have sexual problems. You need to be aware that loss of sex drive is a common problem for people with a chronic illness. If problems with sex are a major concern for you, it may help you to have counselling.

Information and the internet

There is a lot of information about IBS on the internet. Many people with IBS use the internet to communicate and exchange ideas and experiences. At the moment, about 10% of people have regular access to the internet using their own personal computers, and many others can use the internet in public libraries and 'cybercafes' (cafes which have computers you can use to get access to the internet). Over the next few years, most people will be able to use the internet with digital television.

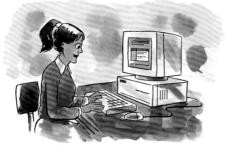

Information on the internet's World Wide Web is contained on webpages. There are three main types of webpage containing information for people with IBS. *The website addresses listed in this section were all correct when this guide was printed.*

Medical webpages

These pages are produced by hospitals or medical charities and contain reliable and often detailed medical information about the disease. They are useful for people who want more information about their illness or to find out about the latest research into aspects of the disease.

Here are some examples of this type of webpage.

http://www.uel.ac.uk/pers/C.P.Dancey/ibs.html

http://www.iffgd.org/

http://www.niddk.nih.gov/health/digest/pubs/irrbowel/irrbowel.htm

http://www.digestivedisorders.org.uk/leaflets/ibs.html

Personal pages

These webpages are usually written by people with IBS who want to share their experiences or communicate with other internet users. Anybody can set up their own webpage. Most of the personal page are genuine attempts by people with IBS to help others by giving advice and letting them know that they are not suffering alone. These webpages may als be used as noticeboards where people can leave messages for other readers.

No two patients have exactly the same symptoms or pattern of disease and some experiences or treatments described by patients may not be relevan to you.

Here are some examples of this type of webpage.

http://www.healingwell.com/ibs/

http://www.ibsgroup.org/

http://www.panix.com/~ibs/

Advertisements

Most webpages directed towards people with IBS ar trying to sell you something. Some of these pages ar obviously advertisements but many appear as perso pages where the writer claims that a certain produc has helped their disease. You should be wary of thes claims of help or cure by these products as they ma not have been tested properly and that is why they are offered over the internet. People with chronic illnesses are often vulnerable and are willing to try

nything that may help their symptoms. If you hear of
product that you think may be useful, try to find out
more about it. A library, pharmacist or health-food
shop may have more information, but please do not
take people's claims or recommendations at face
value. If these products were useful, we would already
be using them.

Take a note of your own favourite websites here.

_____

_____

_____

_____

_____

_____

_____

_____

_____

_____

Recent research in IBS

There has been a great deal of research into IBS in th
past few years. Many of the studies have looked at
possible drug treatments for IBS. These studies show
that certain new drugs may be helpful for different
symptoms of IBS. New drugs are being developed to
control the pain suffered by people with IBS. Other
research is looking at hormones and other chemicals
involved in the way the gut works. Some chemicals
are known to reduce the muscle activity of the colon
and there are others which make the colon less
sensitive. So far, the research has shown that while
these chemicals might be relevant to the symptoms c
IBS, they have not yet been proved to be effective in
people with IBS. There are no signs that a drug will b
found that will cure all the symptoms of IBS.

New techniques are becoming available to researche:
which allow detailed studies to be made on what is
happening to the bodies of people with IBS. These
techniques measure the muscle movements of the gu
and can be used to find out how sensitive the gut is t
pain. Recent research is helping to explain which
parts of the gut contract most in people with IBS.
Research has shown that in people with IBS, certain
parts of the digestive system are very sensitive to
pressure and pain. When more is known about the
action of different parts of the gut and where it goes
wrong in people with IBS, then drugs can be
developed to deal with these problems.

Two new drugs have been developed which may be
helpful for people with IBS. The drugs contain
alosetron and will be launched in the United Kingdo
in early 2001. Later versions of this book will provide
more information and look at the research evidence
for their usefulness

esearchers are also looking at how IBS affects
eople. For example:

- how it affects sleep;

- how it affects people's sex lives;

- when people get pain, in relation to eating and
  opening the bowels;

- whether something that happens in childhood can
  lead to IBS;

- surveys of how long symptoms last and how often
  they come; and

- surveys of how people's daily lives are affected by
  IBS.

ther recent research covers the following theories:

- whether IBS is connected with the menstrual
  cycle;

- whether IBS is inherited;

- whether the anatomy of people with IBS is
  different;

- whether IBS is linked to sexual abuse;

- how IBS is linked to stressful events;

- how IBS is linked to the brain's perception of the
  gut; and

- whether there is a link between food and IBS
  symptoms.

l this research is helping doctors understand what is
ppening to people with IBS, but no one can yet say
actly what causes IBS or when there will be a cure
r IBS.

e do know that if you take control and manage your
S instead of letting it manage you, then you are
ore likely to feel better.

Useful phone numbers and addresses:

IBS Network
Northern General Hospital, Sheffield, S5 7AU
Phone: 0114 2611531

Aromatherapy
To get information about qualified therapists contact:

Aromatherapy Organisation Council,
PO Box 19834, London, SE25 6WF
Phone and Fax : 0181 2517912

Transcendental meditation
Transcendental meditation,
Freepost, London, SW1P 4YY

Yoga
Contact your local health or fitness centre for details
of evening classes

Reflexology
Association of Reflexologists,
27 Old Gloucester Street, London, WC1N 3XX
Phone: 0870 5673320
E-mail: aor@reflexology.org

Acupuncture
The Administrator, British Medical Acupuncture
Society, Newton House, Newton Lane, Whitley,
Warrington, Cheshire, WA4 4JA
Phone: 01925 730727 Fax: 01925 730492

Digestive Disorders Foundation
PO Box 251, Edgware, Middlesex HA8 6HG

*http://www.digestivedisorders.org.uk/leaflets/
ibs.html*

Digestive Disorders Foundation gives information to
anyone with a digestive disorder. It raises money for
research. If you want information please send a
stamped addressed envelope to the address above.

Glossary of medical words

Abdomen - The part of the body below the chest. It contains the digestive organs.

Allergy - A disorder in which the body reacts abnormally to a particular substance. The symptoms are always the same and go away if the substance causing the symptoms is removed.

Anus - The back passage through which faeces leave the body.

Biopsy - A small sample of tissue taken from the lining of the intestine during endoscopy and colonoscopy. It is looked at through a microscope.

Chronic - Long lasting.

Colon - The large intestine where faeces are formed.

Colonoscopy - Passing a long bendy tube through the anus to send images to a video receiver. This is used to examine the whole of the colon.

Duodenum - The first part of the small intestine. The duodenum is connected to the stomach.

Endoscope - An instrument which is used to look inside your body.

Enzyme - A protein that speeds up a biological reaction. Enzymes are vital for the body to work normally.

Faeces - The body's waste - also called stools or motions.

Flatulence - Burping or farting.

Food intolerance - When eating a certain food causes discomfort and illness.

Gastroenterologist - A doctor or a surgeon who is trained to deal with the digestive system.

Gastrointestinal - To do with the digestive system.

Hypersensitive – When the body overreacts to something.

Ileum – The last part of the small intestine. It joins to the colon.

Jejunum – The middle length of the small intestine. It connects the duodenum to the ileum.

Lactase – An enzyme that changes lactose to glucose during digestion.

Lactose – A sugar found in milk or milk products.

Laxative – A drug used to make you empty your bowel.

Mucus – A white slime the intestine produces to help food pass through.

Nutrients – Food which the body needs to grow and work properly.

Oesophagus – The food pipe which connects the mouth to the stomach.

Side effects – Unwanted effects some medicines can have on you.

Sigmoidoscopy (flexible) – A short bendy tube which is passed through the rectum and passes images to a video receiver. It can look into the lower colon.

Sigmoidoscopy (rigid) – Passing a short plastic tube with a light in it, through the anus to look at the rectum.

Stools – The body's waste - also called faeces or motions.

Urgency – The need to go to the toilet immediately.

Useful references

These are examples of some of the books and articles which we used to write this book.

Shirley Price and Len Price. *Aromatherapy for Health Professionals.* Published by Churchill Livingstone, Edinburgh 1995.

Bensoussan A, Talley NJ, Hing M, Menzies R, Guo A, Ngu M. *Treatment of Irritable Bowel Syndrome with Chinese Herbal Medicine.* Journal American Medical Association 1998;280:1585-1589.

Bohmer CJM, Tuynman HARE. *The Clinical Relevance of Lactose Malabsorption in Irritable Bowel Syndrome.* European Journal of Gastroenterology and Hepatology 1996;8:1013-1016.

Collins C. *Yoga: Intuition, Preventive Medicine, and Treatment.* Journal Obstetric Gynecological and Neonatal Nursing 1998;27:563-568.

Klein KB. *Controlled Treatment Trials in the Irritable Bowel Syndrome: A Critique.* Gastroenterolgy 1988;95:232-241.

Knight S. *Use of transcendental meditation to relieve stress and promote health.* British Journal of Nursing 1995; 4:315-318.

Liu JH, Chen GH, Yeh HZ, Huang CK, Poon SK. *Enteric-coated peppermint-oil capsules in the treatment of irritable bowel syndrome: a prospective, randomized trial.* J.Gastroenterol. 1997;32:765-768.

Von Onciul J. *Stress at work.* British Medical Journal 1996;313:745-748.

Whorwell PJ. *Use of Hypnotherapy in Gastrointestinal Disease.* British Journal of Hospital Medicine 1991;45:27-29.

Self-help checklist

Self-help checklist

You may find it helpful to try out different types of self-help treatment and note down how useful they have been to you. You can refer to these notes if your IBS ever becomes a problem in the future. The notes may also help in discussions with your doctor if you need to make an appointment about your IBS. **Fill in the tables below.**

	Date you tried it	Did it help?		Comment
Aromatherapy	/ /	Yes ☐	No ☐	
Yoga	/ /	Yes ☐	No ☐	
Meditation	/ /	Yes ☐	No ☐	
Exercise	/ /	Yes ☐	No ☐	
Join IBS support group	/ /	Yes ☐	No ☐	
Hypnotherapy	/ /	Yes ☐	No ☐	

Self-help checklist

Drugs	have tried	Date	Did they help?		Comment
			Yes	No	
For constipation		/ /	☐	☐	
		/ /	☐ Yes	☐ No	
		/ /	☐ Yes	☐ No	
		/ /	☐ Yes	☐ No	
For diarrhoea		/ /	☐ Yes	☐ No	
		/ /	☐ Yes	☐ No	
		/ /	☐ Yes	☐ No	
For pain		/ /	☐ Yes	☐ No	
		/ /	☐ Yes	☐ No	

Food diary

Write down everything you eat during each day.

	Monday	Tuesday	Wednesday	Thursday	Friday	Saturday	Sunday
Breakfast							
Mid-morning							
Lunch							
Mid-afternoon							

Food diary

	Monday	Tuesday	Wednesday	Thursday	Friday	Saturday	Sunday
Evening meal							
Supper							
Other snacks							
Symptoms							
Possible stresses							